ARTHRITIS AND RHEUMATOLOGY

Arthritis and Rheumatology

My Wonderful Six-Decade Experience

Amazing History, Current Management, Future Outlook

Alfred Becker, MD.

Alfred Becker, MD.
Arthritis and Rheumatology
My Wonderful Six-Decade Experience
Amazing History, Current Management, Future Outlook

Published by Spines
ISBN: 979-8-90223-469-2

Contents

Preface

This book was not written to teach rheumatology in the conventional sense. There are excellent textbooks, clinical guidelines, and review articles that can do a far better job than I ever could do. Nor is this book meant to be a comprehensive or definitive scientific treatise. Much of what we "know" in medicine is provisional, and nowhere is that more evident than in the field of rheumatology.

Rather, these pages are a reflection—sometimes orderly, sometimes meandering—on more than six decades spent caring for patients suffering from arthritis and autoimmune disease. It is an attempt to describe how a field has evolved, often in unexpected ways, and how clinical understanding is shaped as much by uncertainty, observation and humility as by technology and laboratory data.

When I began my medical training, rheumatology was a specialty with few effective therapies and many unanswered questions. Diagnostic tools were limited. We listened carefully, examined patients meticulously, and relied heavily on concentrated observation. Much of what we now take for granted—advanced imaging, sophisticated immunologic assays, targeted biologic therapies—did not exist. Yet patients came, suffered, and trusted us nonetheless.

Over the years, I have watched rheumatology undergo a remarkable transformation. Treatments once considered implausible or even dangerous—gold salts, antimalarials, chemotherapeutic agents, monoclonal antibodies—became cornerstones of care, often discovered through serendipity, false assumptions or entirely unrelated lines of inquiry. At the same time, I have learned that technological progress, for all its merits, carries its own risks. Laboratory tests and imaging studies can inform knowledge, but they cannot replace clinical judgement. Numbers alone do not tell a patient's story.

This book is written for several audiences. Medical students and trainees may find here a perspective that complements formal education—one that emphasizes clinical reasoning, pattern recognition and the importance of admitting what we do not know. Practicing clinicians may recognize familiar frustrations, uncertainties and quiet satisfactions. Patients and caregivers, particularly those living with chronic rheumatic disease, may gain insight into how their illnesses are understood, how treatments are chosen, and why medicine so often proceeds without simple answers.

I have deliberately avoided presenting rheumatologic disease as a collection of isolated joint problems. Over time, it has become clear that most inflammatory arthritic conditions are manifestations of systemic immune dysregulation rather than localized mechanical failure. This realization shaped not only treatment strategies but also the way we speak to patients about their illnesses. Understanding that the immune system can misinterpret one's own tissues as foreign remains one of the most profound—and unsettling—concepts in modern medicine.

Throughout these pages, I have resisted the temptation to smooth over uncertainty. There are many conditions for which we have effective therapies, but little understanding of the root cause of the condition. There are other conditions where we understand the underlying mechanisms in exquisite detail, yet struggle to meaningfully alter the course of disease. Saying "I don't know" has never felt to me a statement of failure; rather, it is often the beginning of honest inquiry.

This book reflects my personal experiences, biases and limitations. It is not meant to establish dogma, promote specific products or predict the future of the field with confidence. If there is a single guiding principle behind these reflections, it is this: progress in medicine depends not only on discovery, but on curiosity, skepticism, compassion, and the willingness to question our own assumptions.

I owe an enormous debt to my teachers, colleagues, and—above all—my patients, who allowed me into their lives during moments of vulnerability and pain. They were my greatest instructors. I am equally indebted to my family, whose patience and support sustained me through a lifetime in medicine.

If this book encourages readers to think more carefully, listen more closely, and remain intellectually humble in the face of complex disease, it will have served its purpose.

Chapter 1

Reflections on a Life in Rheumatology

Having participated in the field of Rheumatology for over six decades, I feel compelled to share some of my inner reflections on this remarkable specialty. This book is not intended to be therapeutic or prescriptive. Nor does it offer guidelines; it is simply a stream of consciousness, a euphoric expression of my lifelong fascination with the conditions that have plagued humankind since antiquity.

Arthritis long predates modern medicine. Paleontologists have identified evidence of inflammatory joint disease in Egyptian mummies. Arthritis is not uniquely human; there is evidence of joint pathology having plagued dinosaurs. Osteoarthritis is common in our familiar animals as well. Many dog owners are aware of arthritic issues in their pets. These observations remind us that rheumatic disease is deeply rooted in life history.

For readers who are interested in finding the sources of these comments, I can suggest some fascinating articles:

A. "3,500-year-old burial of Nubian woman reveals one of world's earliest known cases of rheumatoid arthritis," Jennifer Nalewicki, International Journal of Paleontology, 2/9/24.

B. "The first evidence of osteomyelitis in a sauropod dinosaur," Rodolfo A. Garcia, Ignacio A. Cerda, et al. https://doi.org/10.1111/let.12189, pp. 227–236, Sept. 30, 2016.
C. "Osteoarthritis in dogs: Symptoms, causes," Amanda Simonson, DVM, PetMD 7/1/24.

The language of rheumatology reflects its long history. The Greek word *árthron* means "joint," while *rheuma* in Latin means "flowing," reflecting the ancient belief that illness arose from the flow of humors in bodily fluids. *Lumbago* stems from *lumbus,* meaning "low back," and *inflammation* itself comes from the Latin *inflammare,* to set on fire, aptly describing the heat and pain of swollen joints. The suffix *-itis,* in medical Greek, simply means "inflammation."

Hippocrates believed all disease originated from an imbalance of four humors: blood, black bile, yellow bile and phlegm—a theory later codified by Galen. Treatments were empirical and often imaginative, ranging from garlic and mustard to wine and oils rubbed into sore joints. Willow bark, the precursor of aspirin, became one of humanity's earliest and most enduring attempts to relieve pain.

Beginnings in Syracuse

My earliest memories of medicine date back to my childhood in Syracuse, New York. My father worked tirelessly in a downtown wholesale store while my mother supplemented our income by babysitting. When I became ill, she would place a gentle hand on my forehead to gauge my temperature. If she suspected a fever, she produced a thermometer. If my temperature proved high, I was first prescribed tea with lemon and sugar. When that failed, rock sugar was added—something I doubt one can even find in stores today. If my condition persisted, my mother would summon our family doctor, who made house calls (a concept that today's patients might regard as mythical).

Upon arrival, the doctor was ushered into the dining room, where he was served tea and my mother's incomparable chocolate chip cookies. Only after a discussion of world events and the latest sports scores would he turn to examine me. Wearing his mirror headband, he would instruct me to open my mouth and say "Ahhh." If he then turned to my mother and murmured "Mmm…mmm," I knew my illness was genuine.

He retrieved from his black bag (every doctor had a black bag) a tongue depressor, a cotton swab and a vial of foul-smelling purple liquid. With solemn precision, he applied the swab to my throat. I knew better than to gag, for one stern glance from my mother could communicate, without words, *"Stop being a baby…or else."* (I never dared to reach the "or else" stage.) Remarkably, his treatments always worked. Within a week, I was well again. While my childhood friends dreamed of becoming policemen or firemen, I knew I wanted to be like that doctor—calm, capable, and caring.

The Making of a Doctor

At Syracuse Central High School, I chose to study Latin after learning that physicians once wrote their prescriptions in Latin. I earned a respectable B+, which, I thought, placed me on the right path. I loved science but struggled terribly with mathematics. Fortunately, biology offered me a level of redemption. My fascination with life's mysteries grew, and with it, my determination to become a physician.

I was accepted to the Albert Einstein College of Medicine in its very beginning. I was in the fourth graduating class. The school was so new that tiles were still being laid down as professors lectured. Medical school was rigorous, demanding complete dedication. In those days, diagnostic technology was limited—no echocardiograms, CT scans, MRIs, ultrasound or PET scans. We relied on our ears, eyes and hands: listening attentively, observing carefully, palpating thoughtfully and using a stethoscope, trying to hear what was going on inside the body.

To support myself, I worked in the university's telephone center, operating a switchboard with wires connecting the various medical departments. When all the lights blinked at once, chaos ensued. It was not unusual for me to connect Neurology when someone wanted Urology —a mistake that probably confused more than one caller.

Residency and the Call of Rheumatology

After graduation, I began my internship at Kings County Medical Center in Brooklyn—a city hospital teeming with patients and humanity. Private rooms were rare; patients lay in vast wards of thirty beds or more, and yet, somehow, they healed. The experience was invaluable. The diversity of illness and resilience of patients provided a real education no textbook could equal.

My true maturation as a physician occurred during my residency in Internal Medicine at the University of Pittsburgh. There, under the guidance of extraordinary mentors, I learned not only medicine but compassion, humility and the art of listening. It was during that time that I discovered rheumatology—a field that immediately captivated me. Though our therapeutic options were few, our curiosity was boundless. We sought not only to ease pain but to understand its source.

A Life in Practice

Returning to my alma mater, I completed a fellowship in Rheumatology. In 1965, I opened my first private practice in Rockland County, New York, devoted exclusively to arthritis and rheumatic diseases. There were no board certifications at the time—anyone could claim to be a rheumatologist—but I proudly hung a modest sign: "Practice Limited to Rheumatology and Arthritis." In 1972, the American College of Rheumatology offered board certification, which, as such, rendered me a board-certified rheumatologist.

To my surprise, patients came—and kept coming. Over the years, my wife and I raised five sons, and my professional and personal lives intertwined in meaningful ways. One of my proudest achievements was helping to establish a dedicated Arthritis Unit at the NYS Rehabilitation Center, later given the name of Helen Hayes Hospital, in West Haverstraw, NY—a novel concept at that time. It was a full floor devoted solely to patients with rheumatic diseases, staffed by a multidisciplinary team of orthopedists, physical and occupational therapists, psychologists, nurses and social workers. To my knowledge, it was one of the first and maybe only such comprehensive programs of its kind, and I had the privilege of serving as its Chief of Arthritis Unit for many years. Later, I also provided rheumatology services at the Veterans Hospital in Castle Point, New York—an experience I recall with deep respect and gratitude. The encounter with the patients did not stop when leaving the office.

Chapter 2

Surprising and unexpected encounters over the years as we faced the rheumatic/autoimmune conditions

I never cease to be amazed at how knowledge is gained via peculiar and totally unexpected encounters and happenings. So many things are discovered by chance and occasionally even by false interpretations and assumptions. On the other hand, it is amazing how sophisticated the field of rheumatology has become over the past few decades, so that research and cures are targeted towards the root causes of the condition.

The Golden Age of Gold Treatment

Few remember that gold intramuscular injections once played a major role in treating rheumatoid arthritis. The story began with a mistaken theory that tuberculosis causes arthritis. Since heavy metals were being tested against tuberculosis, gold was tried—and failed to help TB patients. Surprisingly, some patients with rheumatoid arthritis improved dramatically. Thus began the "golden era" of gold injections. At the Hospital for Special Surgery, dosing was refined: typically 50 mg of gold salts intramuscularly monthly after an initial loading phase. For decades, this was considered standard care. This is a glaring example of coming upon a therapy based on a totally false premise, namely that rheumatoid arthritis is caused by tuberculosis. With the advent of a group of therapies called biologics, the treatment with gold therapy essentially disappeared.

The Lowly Aspirin

Everybody is familiar with aspirin. However, the history of this agent is absolutely fascinating. The story relates to an 18th-century English monk by the name of Reverend Edward Stone, who apparently had a tremendous thirst for experimentation and knowledge. History indicates he noticed that the bark of a willow tree contained a bitter-tasting material. We are not absolutely sure of his reasoning. However, in those days, illness was considered to be a result of an imbalance of four humors, outlined as far back as Hippocrates. As far as we know, Stone made a powder out of the willow tree bark and gave it to patients who had a fever and inflammation. He noticed that many of those individuals responded relatively quickly to the powder, to the point that ultimately he documented his findings. In 1763, he wrote a letter to the Royal Society describing his experimentation whereby the powdered extract of a willow tree bark was therapeutic to individuals with fevers and inflammation, titled "An account of the success of the bark of the willow in the cure of agues (the old spelling of aches)". Not much is known about what happened after his letter. In the 1800s, chemists identified the active ingredient causing the fevers to dissipate. The ingredient turned out to be salicylic acid. That product, in and of itself, however, was very corrosive to patients and caused gastrointestinal ill effects. In 1897, Felix Hoffman developed acetyl salicylic acid, which was easier on the stomach. The well-known company, Bayer, copyrighted that agent and called it aspirin.

Aspirin turned out to be a standard of care for numerous inflammatory and feverish conditions. However, nobody understood its mechanism of action and why this acetyl salicylic acid should normalize fevers and inflammation. Have you ever wondered why aspirin lowers a fever of 103° F to a normal of about 98.6°, yet giving aspirin to somebody whose temperature is 98.6° does not cause the temperature to drop to 93.6°?

It's hard to believe that the answer to this puzzle took decades to develop. Sir John Vane discovered that aspirin works by inhibiting an enzyme called cyclooxygenase. Cycloxygenase is involved in the production of prostaglandins, which in turn are responsible for pain, heat and swelling.

I am obviously simplifying Vane's findings. The mechanism of action of aspirin turned out to be extremely complicated. For his revelation, Dr. Vane received the 1982 Nobel Prize in Physiology and Medicine. (As an aside, once you understand prostaglandin inhibition, the answer as to why aspirin lowers high temperature yet does not lower normal temperature becomes clear. Normal individuals simply don't have excess prostaglandins that need to be blocked.) It is of interest that aspirin affects platelets and, as such, is given to individuals who have cardiovascular disease who are at risk of having blood clots.

Non-steroidal anti-inflammatory agents

Once the mechanism of action of aspirin was understood, other agents became available, which also worked on the prostaglandin and inflammatory factors. There are many nonsteroidal anti-inflammatory agents on the market; the choice of which of these agents to take depends to a large extent on subjective criteria of efficacy and patient tolerance, and personal variability. Non-steroidal anti-inflammatory agents do not have a protective effect on the cardiovascular system.

Chemotherapeutic Agents

What I will relate now would sound Neanderthal to current rheumatology students. In the early 1970s, I received a call from a colleague whom I highly respected, who told me that methotrexate is an option for rheumatoid arthritis. I was totally incredulous. Methotrexate was known to be used as chemotherapy for various cancerous illnesses, and I simply could not see how that agent could be used for the treatment of rheumatoid arthritis. Additionally, it was very scary to give cancer chemotherapy for a benign condition such as arthritis. Needless to say, today methotrexate is one of the first-line therapies for rheumatoid arthritis and numerous other rheumatological issues. The dosage has to be individualized and can be given orally or subcutaneously with careful monitoring. At that time, offering methotrexate for a benign condition was totally counterintuitive.

Anti-malarial Agents

Here again was a great surprise. Why would a drug like hydroxychloroquine, also known as Plaquenil, which is used against malaria—a parasite—work for rheumatoid arthritis and other rheumatological conditions? This agent is now also one of the first-line therapies for many rheumatologic issues! Hard to believe that an anti-malaria agent would work in treating rheumatic illness! We now know that the anti-malarials have the capacity to reduce autoantibody-driven inflammation. These drugs have become indispensable in the treatment of rheumatoid arthritis and systemic lupus erythematosus.

Sulfasalazine

Here again came an unexpected therapeutic agent. Why on earth would an agent related to sulfa drugs be a therapeutic agent for rheumatic illness? But it is considered to be one of the first-line drugs for rheumatoid arthritis. The mechanism of action has now been worked out, whereby the sulfasalazine has been shown to inhibit immune activation and inflammatory signaling pathways. How it works was only understood a long time after its efficacy was established.

Tumor Necrosis Factors

The history behind this form of treatment points to the almost comical way therapeutic agents are found. In 1975, a group at Sloan Kettering Institute found a substance that could destroy tumors in mice. They called it tumor necrosis factor (TNF). The word "necrosis" implies cell death. They first thought that this agent could be used to cure cancer. That's where the name tumor necrosis factor came from. This name, in fact, turned out to be a total misnomer, as the factor does not cure tumors. But as is true in so many issues of history, the name stuck.

In the 1980s, it became apparent that the factor that they had called tumor necrosis factor, in fact, was a major driver of inflammation, especially in autoimmune diseases. So, from an initial perception of cancer curing, this group of substances was viewed as a force that creates autoimmune diseases, which are characterized by inflammatory conditions. In the 1980s and 1990s, agents were produced that could block the effect of this tumor necrosis factor. The technical term for these inhibitors is monoclonal antibodies and TNF Inhibitors. This is an example of how a wrong theory ended up being a major player in the treatment of human disease.

The Absolutely Peculiar Name Carried by the Condition of Systemic Lupus Erythematosus—Red Wolf!

If it weren't such a serious illness, the terminology of the word "lupus" would be comical. The term *lupus*, which means "wolf" in Latin, was coined way back when patients with ulcerations in the face were considered to look as if they had been attacked by a wolf. For anyone who would like to see the history, you can find it at Smith, CD, Cyr, M. "The history of lupus erythematosus from Hippocrates to Osler." Rheumatic disease Clinics of North America, 1988, 14; 1/14.

Once the concept of autoimmunity became established in the nineteen hundreds, the search for various targets involving the autoantibodies began in earnest. As we understand it today, in systemic lupus erythematosus, the body attacks its own tissues, causing damage to the patient's own organs and tissues. But the name lupus erythematosus stuck: Red Wolf! This is an ironic reminder that medical language often preserves history more faithfully than accurately.

The Mighty Lymphocyte

It was a long time before we understood this very mighty blood cell. Soon after the discovery of the microscope, a Dutch microscopist, Jan Swammerdam, discovered the presence of red blood cells in the blood, which were then better described by Antony Leeuwenhoek in 1674. In 1840, white blood cells were described and shown to be increased during inflammation. In 1879, Paul Ehrlich classified the white cells into neutrophils, eosinophils, basophils, lymphocytes and monocytes. Platelets were found in the early 1900s.

What is fascinating about the lymphocytes is that they were originally considered to be simply observers, “spectators" in inflammation, and to have no particular function. They were described as having no granules or ability to swallow bacteria and, as such, no importance.

An absolute revolution occurred in the 1950s, when Burnet and Medawar described the role of lymphocytes as reactors when the body was exposed to foreign substances called antigens. In the 1960s, the lymphocytes were described as having two lines of B and T cells. Since that time, we have gained a tremendous understanding of lymphocytes, whereby there are numerous types of T cells and B cells involved in the immune system, with very complicated interactions between various lymphocytes. This new understanding of the lymphocyte has permitted us to understand normal immunity as well as autoimmunity, and to control aberrations in the system via the current biologics and J kinase inhibitors.

When all is said and done, I feel that the lesson to be learned from the above experiences is that medical progress emanates from careful observation, open-mindedness, and recognizing that unexpected outcomes are not uncommon and need to be respected.

CHAPTER 3

TRYING TO UNDERSTAND THE MECHANISMS DRIVING RHEUMATOLOGIC AND ARTHRITIC CONDITIONS

The modern study of arthritis, in my mind, took form with the founding of the Arthritis and Rheumatism Foundation in 1948, which was dedicated to understanding these diseases scientifically and developing effective therapies.

One must understand the absolute crucial need for classification and giving names to categories when trying to confront various illnesses and conditions. I would say that before there is any attempt at understanding and treating a condition, there has to be a dedicated understanding of the condition itself, and as such, a specific name must be given to characterize and differentiate it from all other conditions. Until 1948, musculoskeletal and rheumatic diseases were described by symptoms and did not have a specific characterization. I cannot overemphasize the absolute requirement of the need for specific characterization when studying any medical condition.

From my perspective, the most important element that the Arthritis and Rheumatism Foundation generated was characterizing the various musculoskeletal diseases and ultimately rheumatic conditions by describing the specific nature of each condition. Our understanding of the various rheumatic/musculoskeletal symptoms and conditions can be characterized along five categories:

- Inflammatory
- Degenerative
- Metabolic
- Infectious
- Idiopathic

The inflammatory illnesses

Since the establishment of the Arthritis and Rheumatism Foundation, our perception of rheumatic illness has changed dramatically. As a result, therapeutic intervention has made a quantum leap improvement in the prognosis of the various rheumatic illnesses.

I believe that a major change in perception was achieved when it was understood that rheumatic illness and arthritis are not purely joint diseases. They are manifestations of an internal disease process that frequently presents with joint inflammation. The main essence of the illness, however, is not within the joint but rather within the immune system! I will concentrate initially on the inflammatory illnesses as outlined by the American College of Rheumatology.

Rheumatoid arthritis

The primary concern in this case is to understand that this is not a disease of joints but rather what scientists call systemic illness. What this means is that there is something in the system that is not working right, and in this particular case frequently manifests itself with joint inflammation, redness, heat and pain. However, this condition can affect other organs, such as the lungs, skin and even the cardiovascular system.

The condition is a very complex illness. I will try to make this understandable on a very rudimentary level. In order to understand rheumatoid arthritis more easily, one has to consider our bodies' ability to fight infection and to recognize the fact that in rheumatoid arthritis, the body is turned on to fight what it perceives as a foreign infective invasion when in fact there is no infection. The fact is that the body is actually fighting its own tissues and organs, which gives it the name of an autoimmune disease.

I will review the process of immunity in some very simplistic terms.

For the sake of argument, let's say a person fell and injured their knee, which results in an open wound. This exposed wound area allows bacteria and viruses to invade and attack. They initially attack locally at the point of entry, but subsequently, if uncontrolled, they can attack the entire body. Our body has a system called the immune system, whereby we have the capacity to stop bacteria and viruses. We have given the name "antigen" to the "bad guys"—the bacteria and viruses. (This is intentionally simplified.)

The body responds very quickly by producing molecules that attempt to halt the movement of the bad guys and render them harmless. We give these molecules the name of "antibodies". The process in and of itself is called immunity, meaning that we are attempting to become immune to the bad guys.

How the body creates these antibodies is absolutely amazing. The body is able to make antibodies when it senses that the "bad guys" have attacked. The story is absolutely unbelievable! The antibodies identify the invaders and produce specific antibodies that recognize the specific invaders. The antibodies are configured to attach themselves to the specific invaders, the antigens, which are, as such, neutralized! Once the antibody neutralizes the antigen, a multiplicity of additional defensive events occurs, making sure that the invaders have been stopped. The total result of this "warfare" is manifested as what we call inflammation, in the form of redness, swelling, heat and pain. All of this is the wonderful capacity of the body to recognize the invaders and to try to neutralize them.

Let us imagine a time, however, when the body, for whatever reason, recognizes some of its own tissues as "bad guys." The body responds with an attack, the way it would normally attack an invader. A tremendous response occurs whereby the antibodies and all the associated events that normally respond to an infection attack the body's own tissues. The word that we use to describe this event is autoimmunity. *Auto* is a Greek word that means "self." What the word autoimmunity implies, therefore, is that the body is fighting its own tissues the way it would normally attempt to make the body immune to outside invaders!

In rheumatoid arthritis, the tissues that are most affected with an inflammatory response are the joints. However, other tissues can also be attacked and result in inflammation of the various organs involved. A totally enigmatic finding is that there is a genetic marker, HLA DRB1, which is somehow correlated with rheumatoid arthritis and other rheumatic illnesses.

As of this time, we have not identified the reason why the body would misinterpret itself as a foreign antigen. However, the fact that we do understand what is happening has allowed marvelous therapeutic agents to become available. These agents attempt to modulate and lower the immune response, which in our case is the cause of the damage to the joints and any other organs.

In 1937, a bacteriologist, Erik Waaler, described the phenomenon that the serum of patients with rheumatoid arthritis contained antibodies to other normal antibodies. This offered us a blood test identifying many (but not all) patients who have rheumatoid arthritis. Needless to say, the test was not 100% accurate. However, in addition to the diagnostic tool helping us identify patients with rheumatoid arthritis, it gave us insight into the mechanism of the disease process. The finding was compatible with the idea that in rheumatoid arthritis, there are abnormal antibodies attacking normal tissue and normal antibodies.

This finding opened a hint that the antibodies in the serum of the patients with rheumatoid arthritis attack normal tissues. Here was a clue indicating that in rheumatoid arthritis, the body fights itself as if it were an infection. The term *autoimmunity* was coined. The blood test, with some modifications, has become standard for making the diagnosis of rheumatoid arthritis over the years.

Viewing rheumatoid arthritis as an autoimmune disease was a major game-changer in understanding rheumatoid arthritis. Previously, rheumatoid arthritis was considered an infectious tuberculosis disease, which is why gold was considered a treatment option at a time when gold injections were given for tuberculosis. The prevailing theory at the time was that tuberculosis would respond to gold treatments, and as such, the gold injections would treat rheumatoid arthritis. With the understanding of autoimmunity in rheumatoid arthritis, the whole concept of rheumatoid arthritis being an autoimmune disease was understood to mean that the body is attacking itself. The perception of autoimmunity has been revolutionary because it gave us insight that the enemy in rheumatoid arthritis is not a foreign agent, but rather a misreading of one's own tissues as an enemy. The cause of this misreading still eludes us.

In summary, rheumatoid arthritis is a condition where the body is misinformed and considers its own structures as enemies that need to be attacked.

Systemic lupus erythematosus

This condition is one of the most difficult illnesses to characterize, understand, and get a better handle on its causes and treatments. Given the multiplicity of the presentation of this condition, one cannot help but wonder whether, in fact, everything that we call systemic lupus erythematosus is one and the same disease. Could there be numerous conditions generating all these presentations?

The issue is such that the American College of Rheumatology identified 11 characteristics and manifestations of this disease. An individual who has at least four of those eleven manifestations can then be diagnosed as having systemic lupus erythematosus. The 11 manifestations are described later.

The mere fact that there are so many manifestations of this disease and that there must be a formal count of at least four of those manifestations before systemic lupus erythematosus can be diagnosed indicates how difficult it is to characterize and to study it in depth. At the end of the day, we really have to look at this condition as a generalized autoimmune process affecting a multiplicity of organs and resulting in multiple manifestations.

There appears to be a genetic propensity driving this condition because there are families where multiple members suffer from lupus. It should be said, however, that we really don't have a good handle on the genetic aspect of this disease.

I would like to relate a fascinating case that I had followed in my practice, in which I had a set of identical twins as patients. One of them had classical systemic lupus erythematosus with multiple manifestations. Her twin sister had absolutely no symptoms, but she had extremely high abnormal laboratory tests of ANA, anti-Smith antibody, and anti-double-stranded DNA antibody. I monitored these twins for many decades, and nothing ever changed. The situation was always the same, whereby one of the twins had active disease clinically, while the other did not.

There is no choice but to admit that the root cause(s) and mechanism(s) of systemic lupus erythematosus are still nowhere in sight of understanding. It is clearly an autoimmune disease, as manifested by the fact that there are so many immunological serological markers. But why the disease manifests itself in so many different ways makes the understanding of the real roots and mechanism of action of this condition totally enigmatic.

As such, systemic lupus erythematosus can be viewed as an autoimmune disease with a multiplicity of clinical manifestations.

Scleroderma/systemic sclerosis

The underlying cause of this condition is extremely difficult to establish. There are serological markers of positive ANA, anti-polymerase III, Scl 70, which point to autoimmunity. However, we have absolutely no concept of what drives the body to have manifestations of thickening of the skin, both in terms of local areas and systemic areas. We have no understanding of why there are risks of renal crisis, which can be life-threatening. I have not been able to understand the connection between Raynaud's phenomenon, wherein the fingers and toes show the presence of vascular constriction of whitening, bluish and red colorations, and how those vascular manifestations are related to the abnormal skin process.

Admittedly, there are many theories, but none of these satisfy me. There is a theory that the vascular constriction seen in scleroderma and Raynaud's is what causes the skin to thicken as a result of vascular constriction. I personally don't buy it. When it comes to understanding the underlying causes of diseases involving the rheumatological field, I'm never embarrassed to say "I don't know."

The inflammatory muscle diseases of dermatomyositis, polymyositis and inflammatory muscle disease

We view these conditions as autoimmune inflammatory processes, the cause of which is totally unknown. It is of interest that there is a condition whereby individuals develop an immune-mediated inflammatory muscle disease generated by taking anti-cholesterol statins. What is most intriguing is that these individuals actually have antibodies to the factors that the statins inhibit. Here is an area where we can identify a cause for autoimmunity, whereby the statins generate autoantibodies called HMG-CoA. I can't help but speculate that perhaps there are other, as of yet unknown, stimuli that cause all the known autoimmune diseases.

Vasculitis

This is an array of diseases manifested by numerous findings. It is generally a condition whereby blood vessels become inflamed. What is very interesting is that there are some vasculitides that result from hepatitis B and some from hepatitis C. Are we absolutely sure that the rest of the vasculitides conditions are not also caused by some agent whose identity we have not found in this day and age? In summary, this is a group of conditions whereby numerous blood vessels of various sizes get inflamed and can affect a variety of organs.

Polymyalgia rheumatica

There are a number of highly speculative theories as to the cause or causes of this condition, which manifests itself with severe musculoskeletal pain, stiffness, and occasionally a very serious complication of temporal arteritis, which can result in visual loss. It generally does not cause permanent joint damage. What is interesting is that the condition appears to be coming in clusters, especially after winter. Is there something in the environment, such as a virus, that generates this condition? Another puzzle is that the condition has a positive correlation with a genetic marker called HLA DRB1, which is also prevalent in rheumatoid arthritis. I can only speculate that some biological agent (perhaps a virus?) in the environment, especially after the winter, creates this particular condition that sets off the immune response, causing musculoskeletal pain and even the dreaded complication of temporal arteritis.

Polymyalgia rheumatica is, as such, a non-crippling musculoskeletal condition characterized by joint pain and stiffness that has the potential of affecting the temporal artery with the dreaded potential possibility of causing visual impairments. For reasons that are not clear, it can come in clusters after the winter, which makes an outside environmental factor a highly speculative rationale to explain this condition.

Psoriatic arthritis

We don't have a clue as to what the underlying issues that cause this condition are. There are many clinical expressions that create an array of speculation. This condition is frequently found in conjunction with a positive genetic marker called HLA B27. Surprisingly, the arthritic manifestations can sometimes develop many years after the onset of the psoriasis. Why did the arthritis wait so long? Psoriatic arthritis has manifestations that are different from classical rheumatoid arthritis. The joints involved, unlike rheumatoid arthritis, are frequently non-symmetrical, which means that they can affect one side of the body without necessarily affecting the other side. It is also of interest that the condition frequently affects the toes.

Additionally, there is a strange correlation between inflammatory arthritis of the spine and psoriasis and psoriatic arthritis. Can anybody make sense of all this? I do not think so at this time. But in the future, perhaps somebody will be able to put all this together and give us an understanding of the root cause of this condition.

Psoriatic arthritis is a joint and skin condition. The two conditions do not necessarily have to occur at the same time. The condition can be associated with arthritis in the spine in certain instances.

Juvenile idiopathic arthritis

What is so enigmatic in this case is the fact that there are so many children for whom the condition ultimately remits, many times spontaneously. What is the root cause of this condition? We haven't got a clue.

This is a condition affecting young people whose prognosis is totally unpredictable. It needs to be treated quickly and aggressively to prevent joint and growth damage. The mechanism generating this condition in children is totally shrouded in mystery.

Ankylosing spondylitis/Non-radiographic axial spondyloarthropathy

What characterizes this group of conditions is a frequent association with a genetic marker of HLA B27. How that specific gene generates autoimmunity against spinal tissue is totally unknown. This condition has to be differentiated from a common spinal disc disease, which is a frequent condition and has a totally different underlying process.

Ankylosing spondylitis is an autoimmune spinal inflammatory disease affecting the spine, unlike disc disease, which is what we call a degenerative process rather than an inflammatory disease. A closely related condition is non-radiographic spondyloarthritis, which carries many of the clinical characteristics of Ankylosing Spondylitis with normal X-rays.

Inflammatory eye disease

These are considered autoimmune diseases, as manifested by the fact that there are serological markers such as ANA positivity. The fact that there is a propensity for HLA B27 positivity makes speculation only more difficult as to why there would be a genetic driver for autoimmunity.

This condition is treated in conjunction with ophthalmology.

Sjogren's syndrome

This condition is characterized by dry eyes and a dry mouth. The issue is complicated because there are many individuals who just feel that they have dry eyes and/or a dry mouth, and don't really have this condition. There are specific tests that can help us make the diagnosis. We can literally measure the amount of tears an individual produces with a test called a Schirmer's test. We can measure the amount of saliva an individual produces per given time with a test called Sialometry. There are abnormal blood tests called SS-A and SS-B antibodies. Generally, the patients will have elevated inflammatory markers of ESR and CRP. The disease is essentially an autoimmune disease affecting the salivary and lacrimal (tear-producing) glands. Just as is true of so many rheumatic illnesses, Sjogren's has a systemic element, whereby other organs can be involved. Sjogren's can involve the lungs, kidneys, joints, skin and even the nervous system. Fatigue is another common complaint. These people tend to have a propensity for dental cavities and, on rare occasions, lymphomas. Occasionally, a salivary gland biopsy will be ordered.

Sjogren's is a condition generally involving dry eyes and dry mouth. However, other manifestations of this disease can occur and need to be evaluated and monitored carefully.

In summary, the above entities are considered to be autoimmune entities. The theory at this time is that there's some unknown cause(s) that makes the body's defense system misinterpret its own tissues as an enemy entity, and the immune system attacks its own organs.

Degenerative joint diseases/Osteoarthritis

The names of this category, degenerative arthritis and osteoarthritis, are, as far as I'm concerned, totally erroneous and irrelevant. I do not believe that the various entities that fall under the term degenerative joint disease are a result of a degenerative process.

Admittedly, we don't really know what causes certain joints to develop arthritic changes. What is most puzzling is that an individual may have severe arthritic changes in the left hip and none in the right hip, or in the knee and nothing in other joints. Not every football player ends up with joint disease. Yet, just watch a football player and note the constant and recurrent impact on the joints! Many patients have been sedentary all their lives and develop arthritic changes, which we now call degenerative arthritis. In addition, they may have only one single joint involved, which certainly does not make the term degenerative arthritis logical, because why wouldn't other joints be subject to the degeneration as well? The term osteoarthritis is also misleading. The word *osteo* means bone, whereas the actual pathology in these conditions resides in the cartilage.

I would not be surprised if, ultimately, we will identify a genetic mechanism that renders cartilage susceptible to damage. Additionally, I would not be surprised if, in the future, some unknown biological agent whose name we haven't even discovered at this time is shown to cause these changes. What this discussion does identify, however, is how little we really understand about the cause of these conditions, which go under the name of osteoarthritis.

During my professional experience over the years, the condition has had a dramatic therapeutic paradigm. I must admit that when I started out as a rheumatologist in the 1960s, when the hip didn't work, you were considered an invalid. The idea of putting in a new joint (which technically is called Joint Replacement or arthroplasty) was absolutely preposterous. How could you possibly put a new joint into a person?!

In this day and age, joint replacement has become progressively more efficient, and people's lives have been ameliorated dramatically in terms of function and pain. Ultimately, however, I'm looking for the time when we can actually repair the damaged cartilage and even more hopeful is the possibility that the cartilage will never be damaged with the appropriate preventive therapeutic intervention.

Deep down in my mind, I believe that the root cause of the so-called degenerative arthritis is, at this time, totally unknown. I do not hold that it is a manifestation of wear and tear or trauma, although these may contribute to the condition. Somewhere along the line, I believe we will find an agent that attacks cartilage and causes the joint changes which in this day and age we call degenerative arthritis, when in fact it is probably a reactive condition to an underlying agent. But who knows!

Metabolic arthritis

There are numerous metabolic abnormalities that cause joint damage. The two most common metabolic entities are gout and pseudogout.

The causes of these conditions emanate from the presence of crystals in the joints, which can be identified in the joint fluid. The fluid is called synovial fluid. Every joint has a small amount of synovial fluid, whose purpose is to lubricate the joint so it can move effectively. When there is inflammation, excessive fluid may develop, which we technically call joint effusion and colloquially a swollen joint.

An individual who has an attack of gout or pseudogout will have inflammation in the joint. The synovial fluid can be removed both to relieve pain and pressure, and for diagnostic purposes to exactly identify the cause of the inflammation. In gout and pseudogout, crystals can be seen under the microscope within the fluid.

The presence of the crystals sets off a response by the body's blood cells, which tries to eliminate the crystals and, in some cases, actually tries to swallow and digest them. However, the cells do not have the capacity to digest these crystals. The crystals themselves, when swallowed by the blood cells, can cause the cell to rupture, which in turn causes more inflammation, heat and pain.

Gout has been plaguing mankind for centuries. There is a multiplicity of legends pointing to gouty attacks in the ancient world. Alexander the Great is supposed to have had gouty attacks. It should be noted that he is known to have loved alcohol.

When you look under the microscope at the removed synovial fluid in cases of crystal synovitis, you can actually see crystals under the microscope. The two main forms of crystals are uric acid crystals and calcium pyrophosphate crystals.

Interestingly, these two types of crystals have different shapes under the microscope, whereby the uric acid crystals are needle-like, while the crystals of pseudogout are rhomboid-shaped. It is amazing to see the reaction of the body to these crystals under the microscope, when the white blood cells try to swallow the crystals in an attempt to dissolve them. Unfortunately, the crystals do not yield to those cells and, in fact, damage them, whereby there is more inflammation being generated in the joint. Gout and pseudogout can be extremely painful.

Infectious arthritis

Fortunately, we don't see infectious arthritis frequently. Before pasteurization of milk became mandatory in the United States, tuberculosis hip disease was not uncommon. Individuals would drink raw milk, which could have contained tuberculosis bacteria. Tuberculosis would affect the intestines and, in turn, eventually rupture into the hip joints. We simply do not see that in this day and age. The most important component of infectious arthritis, if and when it should occur, is not to miss the diagnosis. A high index of suspicion needs to be maintained whenever there is an inflamed joint with no specific explanation. Once the diagnosis is established, therapeutic intervention is usually effective. However, there are times when treatment is very difficult. This can occur especially when there is a history of previous surgical intervention, such as joint replacement. Infections affecting such joints are much harder to treat. Overall, most commonly, infectious arthritis can be treated effectively. The trick is to make the diagnosis quickly before permanent damage Will have occurred.

The issue of Lyme disease, which really is not an infectious disease, will be discussed later.

Idiopathic arthritis

This is a group of conditions that injects humility into every physician. We always have to admit that there are situations that don't fit into our understanding in terms of cause or therapy. Sometimes, with greater technology and simply over time, the nature of these conditions becomes more apparent, understandable and treatable. I don't believe there are any rheumatologists who can honestly say that they understand 100% of all cases that come through the door. It is important to keep in mind that with effort and patience, perhaps the puzzle can ultimately be solved.

What comes to my mind is the story of Lyme disease. In 1975, a woman in Lyme, Connecticut, was told that her child had juvenile rheumatoid arthritis. She was astute, however, and noted that there were other children in the area, all of whom had what they called juvenile rheumatoid arthritis. She recognized that the density of cases in her neighborhood was just too great, and therefore, suspiciously high, because juvenile rheumatoid arthritis is, fortunately, a rare disease. She was persistent and looked for a cause. The cause was ultimately found by Dr. Willy Burgdorfer, who found that neighborhood ticks were spreading the condition. The ticks were carrying bacteria called spirochetes, which, in turn, caused Lyme disease. The children in the neighborhood did not have juvenile idiopathic arthritis. In all fairness, the credit for the discovery of the tick-borne nature of this condition should have gone to the mother, whose persistence ultimately identified the underlying nature of this condition. The puzzle was finally solved. The kids in her neighborhood did not have a rheumatological entity. Because the ticks were identified as coming from Lyme, Connecticut, the condition is therefore called Lyme disease.

As long as we are honest enough to admit that we don't know everything, there is hope for further understanding of the numerous conditions whose etiology and therapy are still unknown.

Fibromyalgia/Chronic Fatigue

This is one of the most frustrating conditions, both in terms of the patients and the healthcare provider. Initially, it was considered to be an imaginary, emotional condition with no objective cause or findings. All laboratory tests and imaging studies are, almost by definition, negative.

We now recognize that, in fact, the condition is a true and frequently debilitating condition manifested by diffuse musculoskeletal pain, cognitive changes, emotional mood issues, "brain fog" and severe fatigue. No specific therapeutic intervention exists. There are medications on the market approved by the FDA for the fibromyalgia condition. However, their efficacy remains to be improved. The most important element of this condition on the part of the health care provider is to recognize the authenticity of the symptoms and to work with the patient with supportive care, understanding of the condition, and hoping that someday a specific cause for this condition will be identified and a specific therapeutic intervention will be available.

I would like to add that the American College of Rheumatology does recognize this condition as a true medical entity that needs to be treated with respect. (I hate to admit it. However, it had not been uncommon in the past to tell the patient, "It's all in your head. Try to get over it.")

Chapter 4

The wonders and potential pitfalls of our current diagnostic tools

The past decades have seen an amazing array of diagnostic tools that can identify rheumatic illness, evaluate the efficacy of therapeutic intervention, and give a prognosis for individual cases. However, before we look into the specific diagnosis tools, it should be noted that there are some very serious issues that need to be addressed when it comes to evaluating the results of the diagnostic tests.

It is absolutely imperative to look at the entire clinical picture. There is a total need for the provider to take an intensive clinical history, perform a thorough physical examination, and do laboratory testing, as well as imaging studies, before coming to a specific diagnosis. Merely relying on a positive blood test or imaging study is simply inappropriate. It is imperative to evaluate the entire picture before coming to a conclusive recommendation and analysis.

The other issue that needs to be addressed is the fact that numerous clinicians have offered access to laboratory and imaging test results to their patients via the internet and digital websites. From my perspective, laboratory testing and imaging studies should be directed to the patients solely by the healthcare provider. I do not believe that exposing the patient to information without explanation is appropriate. I will relay a true, specific case to you. The patient had been seeing me for decades for rheumatoid arthritis. One day, she came into the office to say goodbye to me because she was convinced that she was about to part from this world. "I am going to die." In questioning her, it turned out that her primary physician had a system whereby the patient can see their laboratory tests immediately via a website. The patient noticed a multiplicity of results that were flagged and labeled as abnormal by the website. She was convinced that, given the multiplicity of abnormalities, she was about ready to depart this world. When I looked at the results, it became apparent that while the computer did flag abnormalities, the results in and of themselves were not clinically relevant to create the situation of panic generated by the information. In retrospect, the story may appear comical. From my perspective, however, this individual underwent tremendous emotional stress, totally unnecessarily, because she was not given a professional evaluation and explanation for the laboratory tests. As such, I feel very strongly that direct contact between the healthcare provider and the patient is imperative when discussing any testing.

On the other side of the coin, the availability of the multiplicity of testing devices and techniques has had an explosive opening to view diagnosis, prognostication and treatment. This is a tool that is still constantly progressing. We have laboratory testing that we never had previously, imaging techniques that are currently and constantly improving, and ultrasound, all of which give us the power to understand and hopefully treat human illness.

As is true in all of life, one has to use knowledge in a rational and appropriate way.

Laboratory and imaging testing tools:

Before starting this discussion, I feel that I have to make several important points. Laboratory tests are powerful but not ultimate diagnostic tools. The fact that we have the capability of ordering serologic testing has changed rheumatology dramatically. The rheumatoid factor, antinuclear antibody (ANA), anti-dsDNA, complement levels, and inflammatory markers, which measure the level of inflammation in the body, such as ESR and CRP, give us tools that offer extreme clarity. But you have to be careful because they can also result in ambiguities. No test in rheumatology is entirely specific. Rheumatoid factors can be positive in chronic infection, malignancy and even in healthy elderly individuals. ANA positivity is common in the general population and meaningless as an isolated finding. On the other hand, patients with unequivocal autoimmune disease may have normal laboratory results, especially early in their illness.

I also feel compelled to make a statement about ordering too many unnecessary tests. Ordering tests indiscriminately generates false positives, anxiety and diagnostic confusion. A positive result divorced from clinical context is not insight; it is noise. I also need to say something about imaging studies. Imaging has advanced dramatically. Ultrasound and MRI now reveal synovitis, bone marrow edema, and erosions long before they are visible on plain radiographs. These tools have tremendous value, especially in early inflammatory arthritis. But we can never forget that imaging abnormalities and findings do not always translate into greater understanding. Imaging can detect abnormalities whose clinical significance is uncertain. Degenerative changes, incidental findings, and age-related alterations are frequently mistaken for disease. The risk is overdiagnosis—treating images rather than patients.

I hate to sound pedantic, but I can't start talking about diagnostic tools before making the following honest assessment. In rheumatology, diagnosis is a process—one that unfolds over time, shaped by observation, reflection and humility.

Rheumatoid Arthritis

Here again, I cannot overemphasize the need to look at the entire patient rather than being focused on laboratory tests.

The classical tests for rheumatoid arthritis are the Rheumatoid Factor and CCP (Cyclic citrullinated peptide) antibodies. It should be noted that there is a significant proportion of individuals who carry a diagnosis of seronegative rheumatoid arthritis, for whom these factors are negative. As such, these tests need to be considered as a piece of evidence but not absolute markers for the presence or absence of this disease.

Major diagnostic tools in evaluating the presence and

level of active inflammatory disease are the ESR and CRP (erythrocyte sedimentation rate and C-reactive protein). These can be viewed as thermometers of the level of inflammatory condition at the time of evaluation, giving us a digital number reflecting the level of activity of the condition. The provider will frequently order additional tests, particularly looking for anemia, which occurs in a significant proportion of rheumatoid patients. There will be Baseline Laboratory Testing in preparation for possible therapeutic intervention. If there are physical findings of concern, X-rays and/or ultrasound may be ordered to identify physical joint abnormalities or damage. In certain circumstances where there is suspicion of extra-articular (issues outside of the joints) involvement, further testing may be ordered. Finally, laboratory tests will be ordered in search of the presence of additional diseases. At the end of the day, this paradigm of findings should identify the condition, its severity and its prognosis.

Systemic Lupus Erythematosus

Establishing the diagnosis of systemic lupus erythematosus is a true challenge. The American College of Rheumatology has listed clinical and immunological criteria to make the diagnosis. As mentioned previously, there are 11 possible manifestations that can occur and need to be evaluated. The patient who has four or more of the 11 criteria is considered to have a positive diagnosis for systemic lupus erythematosus.

As far as laboratory tests are concerned, diagnosis

requires a positive ANA at a titer of at least 1:80. The presence of anti-Smith and anti-double-stranded DNA is very important, with a specificity of 97% for lupus. However, the sensitivity of having a positive test is only 70% in the anti-DNA test and only 20 to 30% in the anti-Smith test. What this means, therefore, is that there are patients who have the disease despite having negative tests.

Numerous tests are ordered in order to get a better insight into the severity of the disease, prognosis and recommendations for therapy. A laboratory test that will frequently be ordered is anti-phospholipid antibodies, also known as anticardiolipin, or Lupus anticoagulant. Their presence indicates a risk for blood clots, known as thrombosis. Serum complement levels are ordered because they are a harbinger of flare-ups of lupus before the flare-up. CBC is looked at for the possibility of anemia, low white counts, and low platelets. Kidney functions, including urinalysis looking for abnormalities such as protein, are evaluated to search for potential kidney involvement of lupus. Under certain circumstances, a kidney biopsy may be required to characterize the nature of the kidney disease.

Scleroderma/Systemic Sclerosis

I would say this is one of the least understood autoimmune diseases. The diagnosis depends mostly on the patient's history and physical examinations. There are, however, laboratory tests that are frequently positive in this condition. Scl 70 antibodies are often found in these conditions, and positive ANA, with what is called a speckled pattern, is frequently found. There will be a search for anti-centromere antibodies. There are other markers that are evaluated, including anti-Th/To Antibodies, which are associated with lung disease. Imaging studies of the lungs searching for interstitial lung disease, unfortunately, a common complication, are ordered routinely. Kidney functions will be evaluated for possible kidney involvement.

Dermatomyositis/Polymyositis

This condition involves the muscles, and the laboratory tests focus on muscle enzymes, such as CPK and aldolase, which search for leakage of the enzymes from damaged muscles. A serious complication of damaged muscles is the presence of an elevated myoglobin level, which can result in kidney failure. The possibility of drug-induced muscle inflammation, especially the statins, is imperative to be considered when this condition begins.

The laboratory tests that I look for in this condition are the anti-Jo1 antibodies. A group of antibodies called anti-synthetase antibodies is also utilized to better understand the various manifestations of this condition. Muscle biopsies, EMG and nerve conduction studies are possible diagnostic studies performed in this condition when deemed warranted. Autoimmune markers, such as ANA, will frequently be positive, pointing to the autoimmunity of inflammatory muscle disease. Cancer screening is appropriate given the possibility of underlying cancer associated with these myopathies, especially dermatomyositis.

Vasculitis

This is a group of inflammatory conditions that involves numerous organs by affecting blood vessels. The choice of laboratory tests in this case is very individualized. Inflammatory markers of ESR and CRP are mandatory. A laboratory test called ANCA, which stands for anti-neutrophil cytoplasmic antibody, is consistent with a condition called granulomatosis with polyangiitis. Kidney functions are evaluated. These conditions are occasionally associated with other autoimmune processes, which results in being called overlap conditions, pointing to the multiplicity of the manifestations in this one patient. As such, ANA and other autoimmune antibodies are searched for. Surprisingly, hepatitis C and hepatitis B can also be associated with these vasculitides syndromes. Cryoglobulins are searched for, especially in hepatitis C infections. Basic testing is performed initially in order to get a better understanding of the general health of the individual. Individualization is absolutely imperative in this set of conditions, given the multiplicity of their manifestations.

Polymyalgia rheumatica

This is a condition that affects older adults, generally above the age of 50. The greatest threat in this instance is the development of what is called temporal arteritis, also called giant cell arteritis, which can, on occasion, result in visual loss. The laboratory tests that are almost invariably positive are the inflammatory markers of ESR and CRP. There are no specific laboratory tests pointing to this condition. The diagnosis depends mostly on the history of diffuse musculoskeletal pain and stiffness. Pain over the temporal artery alerts the provider to consider temporal arteritis. When suspicion of temporal arteritis (giant cell arteritis) is raised, a temporal artery biopsy is required for determination. Ultrasound of the temporal artery may also help in the diagnosis of temporal arteritis and, in some cases, may obviate the need for biopsy.

Psoriatic arthritis

This condition behaves differently from classical rheumatoid arthritis and is frequently associated with psoriasis, although there are situations where the psoriasis will occur years after the onset of the arthritic manifestations. The laboratory tests that are called for are the inflammatory markers of ESR and CRP. It is occasionally associated with a genetic marker called HLA B27. The rheumatoid factor and CCP are usually negative. Rarely, there will be an elevated uric acid level, which reflects the hyperactive skin turnover. An ultrasound and

MRI of the joints may be ordered to document inflammatory elements and/or the presence of erosions. Nevertheless, differentiating psoriatic arthritis from classical rheumatoid arthritis may be difficult. With the availability of biologics, it is important to make the diagnosis correctly because biologics for rheumatoid arthritis are frequently different from the biologics of psoriatic arthritis.

Juvenile idiopathic arthritis

This unfortunate condition affecting young people has an interesting history. Initially, it was called juvenile rheumatoid arthritis. As we understood this condition and evaluated it more closely, it became apparent that, in fact, this condition is not just rheumatoid arthritis affecting children but rather an entity unto itself. There was therefore a change in its name to juvenile idiopathic arthritis.

Currently, the disease affects individuals before the age of 16, and the symptoms must last at least 6 weeks in order to qualify for that diagnosis. The actual classification will be dealt with later. As far as laboratory tests go, the ANA is frequently positive. Rheumatoid Factor and anti-CCP are usually negative. ESR and CRP are variable in terms of their positivity in this condition. Of interest is the fact that the ferritin level is elevated in some of these conditions.

Ultrasound and MRI evaluations will show excessive fluid (effusions), inflammation (synovitis), and possible erosions. A form of juvenile arthritis called Still's disease is characterized by fever, rash, joint pain, sore throat, muscle pain, fatigue, and may result in inflammation of the heart and lungs, and the enlargement of the liver. Fortunately, this is a rare condition. No specific laboratory tests exist to make that diagnosis. Rather, the diagnosis is made on clinical grounds and manifestations.

Ankylosing spondylitis

This is a condition that affects the spine and, occasionally, joints. As far as laboratory tests are concerned, there is a high incidence of positive HLA B27 genetic markers. Inflammatory markers of ESR and CRP are frequently elevated. The rheumatoid factor and anti-CCP are negative. The patients frequently have pain over the sacroiliac joints. The diagnosis depends mostly on imaging studies. X-rays of the sacroiliac joints and the spine will frequently provide the diagnosis. MRIs of the spine and sacroiliac joints will frequently show inflammation or sclerosis.

Non-radiographic Axial Spondyloarthritis

This is a relatively recently recognized entity that carries many but not all features of ankylosing spondylitis. Laboratory tests are frequently positive for HLA B27, and elevated ESR and CRP. By its very nature, X-rays are generally inconclusive. The diagnosis, however, can be made on the basis of an MRI, which shows inflammation in the sacroiliac joints. Overall, however, the diagnosis depends on the clinical manifestations described by the patient.

Episcleritis, Uveitis, Iritis

These are serious complications of various rheumatic diseases. The diagnosis is generally made by the ophthalmologist. Laboratory tests are frequently positive for ANA, elevated ESR, and elevated CRP. HLA B27 is associated in some cases. There are numerous underlying conditions that manifest themselves with inflammation in the eyes. Because of its inflammatory nature, this condition can be considered autoimmune. Involvement of ophthalmology is imperative in these cases.

Crystal synovitis (gout and pseudogout)

The most definitive test is the analysis of the synovial fluid in search of crystals. In gout, the microscopic evaluation of synovial fluid will reveal needle-like crystals that are actually swallowed by the white blood cells. In pseudogout, we see rhomboid-shaped crystals that are made of calcium pyrophosphate.

Laboratory tests that are crucial in this instance search for elevations in serum uric acid. The elevations in the serum uric acid level could be genetic, dietary, metabolic or caused by medications. It must be kept in mind that uric acid crystals can embed themselves in the kidneys and cause kidney stones with potential severe clinical manifestations.

Infectious arthritis

One must always be alert to the possibility of an underlying infectious agent when dealing with inflamed joints. The diagnosis in these instances is invariably done by culturing the appropriate tissues and synovial fluid.

Sjogren's syndrome

There are some relatively specific tests when it comes to Sjogren's syndrome. Tests pointing to this condition are the SS-A and SS-B antibodies and, occasionally, a salivary gland biopsy. Because of the inflammatory nature of this condition, ESR and CRP are frequently elevated. Ophthalmologists can measure tear flow with objective means. After all is said and done, the patients' complaints are the most convincing diagnostic tools because, subjectively, they have dry eyes and a dry mouth.

Fibromyalgia/chronic fatigue syndrome

This diagnosis relies almost completely on the lack of objective abnormalities in laboratory testing and imaging studies. There are numerous subjective manifestations and descriptions, including diffuse musculoskeletal pain, severe fatigue, mood changes and cognitive issues. We generally rely on the chronicity, consistency and credibility of these self-reported symptoms.

CHAPTER 5

TAKING A GOOD HISTORY—HOW RHEUMATIC MANIFESTATIONS ARE DESCRIBED, EVOLVE, AND MAY SIGNAL SPECIAL CONCERN

In plain terms, understanding any medical condition begins with taking a careful and thoughtful history. More often than not, the diagnosis is already present within the patient's narrative—if one listens closely enough. In rheumatology, this is particularly true. Laboratory studies and imaging can refine or support a diagnosis, but they rarely replace the story itself. This chapter reviews how major rheumatic conditions typically present, how they evolve over time, and which features should alert the clinician to potentially serious complications

Rheumatoid arthritis

The disease is generally progressive, starting with some very minor musculoskeletal symptoms of pain and joint stiffness. If an individual describes that they just got up one morning with severe rheumatic symptoms, the diagnosis of rheumatoid arthritis is probably not the correct one. Rheumatoid arthritis most frequently affects the joints symmetrically. This means that the condition affects both sides of the body generally; for example, both wrists or both feet, which represent symmetrical manifestations. It is of interest that rheumatoid arthritis generally does not affect the DIP joints of the hands (the small joints of the fingers which are furthest away from the body). This is a useful diagnostic tool to differentiate rheumatoid arthritis from osteoarthritis. One of the most common manifestations of rheumatoid arthritis is morning stiffness. The duration of the morning stiffness is frequently used as a marker for the severity of the disease. Given the systemic nature of this condition, fatigue, malaise and weight loss are not uncommon.

Systemic lupus erythematosus

This is a challenging condition to diagnose because of its multiplicity of potential manifestations. In fact, the difficulty of making a diagnosis was tackled by the American College of Rheumatology, whereby they listed 11 manifestations of disease and required four of those to be positive in order for the diagnosis of systemic lupus erythematosus to be considered as established. The manifestations are:

1. Malar rash: This is a characteristic rash on the face over the nasal area, which has also been called a butterfly rash because of its distribution.
2. Discoid rash: This is a scaly, scarring rash. The diagnosis is generally made by a dermatologist.
3. Photosensitivity: a skin rash that results from exposure to sunlight (In 1972, Henrietta Aladjem, who had systemic lupus

erythematosus, wrote a book called "The Sun Is My Enemy. One Woman's Victory Over a Mysterious and Dreaded Disease.")

4. Ulcers in the nose or mouth.
5. Tenderness and swelling of at least two joints.
6. Inflammation in the chest resulting in pericarditis and/or pleuritis: This diagnosis is generally established by imaging studies, but depends to a large extent on the description of pain in the chest upon deep breathing.
7. Abnormal urinary findings of excessive protein or abnormal findings on laboratory microscopic evaluation, called casts.
8. Abnormal neurological conditions of seizures and psychosis.
9. Abnormal laboratory tests of anemia, low white counts or low platelets
10. Abnormal laboratory tests of positive anti-dsDNA, anti-Smith antibodies and positive lupus anticoagulant, also known as antiphospholipid antibodies.
11. Positive ANA

What this tells me is that when taking a history, you have to expect that the manifestations of lupus are extremely variable and depend on at least four clinical manifestations.

Scleroderma/Systemic Sclerosis

In this condition, the patient's history will generally point to the diagnosis very quickly. Changes in the skin texture are very noticeable to the patient. They will describe a thickening of their skin. The term sclerosis implies hardening. The reason that scleroderma and systemic sclerosis are listed together is that the conditions manifest themselves with hardening of the skin. There are two types of hardening of the skin described, which are essentially totally different from each other.

Localized scleroderma: This is a condition where the only involvement of the condition is the skin and its underlying tissues, but there is no indication of internal organ involvement. Amongst these conditions, there are two types of manifestations.

Morphea: These are localized thickenings of the skin. Generally, the ANA is negative, which is a manifestation of the localized nature of this condition, as opposed to being a generalized systemic disease. A peculiar aspect of these conditions is that they are occasionally what we call self-limited and may stabilize after 3 to 5 years. Unfortunately, whatever damage they did is permanent. However, there may be no progression to a more systemic disease.

Systemic Sclerosis: This is a generalized systemic disease involving hardening of the skin, inflammation of the blood vessels, and it can involve the lungs, heart and kidneys. Frequently, the patient will describe whitening, bluishness and redness of the fingers, which is called Raynaud's phenomenon, even before the condition manifests itself. Skin thickening usually starts in the fingers and may progress. Calcium deposits can be found in the skin, ulcerations are found in the fingers, and frequently, dilated blood vessels called telangiectasia will be seen on the chest. These are frequently the descriptions revealed by the patient. When there is lung involvement, frequently described by the patient as having a cough or shortness of breath, imaging studies will show abnormalities called interstitial lung disease, which represents scarring of the lungs. Scleroderma can involve the gastrointestinal tract with a characteristic change in its motility, which can be documented with imaging studies. The patient may describe numerous symptoms with reference to their eating habits and bowel characteristics. One of the most threatening complications of this disease is a condition called renal crisis, whereby uncontrolled blood pressure becomes life-threatening. When the condition involves the heart, cardiac rhythm issues may be reported. There may also be symptoms described compatible with the presence of heart failure.

Raynaud's phenomenon: This condition can vary from just being a nuisance to actual ulcerations, which may require beta blocking medications, nitroglycerin and occasionally even surgical sympathectomies. The manifestations described by the patient are whitening, turning bluish and finally redness of the fingers and toes when exposed to cold. Emotional stress can also trigger the manifestations.

Dermatomyositis/Polymyositis/Inflammatory muscle diseases

This is a group of rheumatological entities wherein the body attacks the muscles on an autoimmune basis.

Dermatomyositis: The patient will describe some distinctive skin findings that initially affect the areas over the small joints of the hands. There are also skin problems involving the elbows, ankles and knees. There is a characteristic discoloration around the eyes called heliotropic rash. There are also characteristic skin rashes over the chest, in what is called a V sign distribution, and skin changes called telangiectasia—dilated blood vessels seen through the skin with the appearance of a spider web. The patient will frequently volunteer this information, but the questions still have to be asked pointedly.

The muscle manifestations of this illness show themselves as painful muscles and muscle weakness, whereby the patient may describe difficulties getting out of a chair or climbing stairs. There are individuals in whom the muscles are not affected, and the skin manifestations correlate with this illness. This is called amyopathic dermatomyositis, which obviously is a funny name for this condition, meaning essentially non-muscle disease. Myopathies (muscle diseases) need to be looked at as a systemic generalized illness that can affect the lungs, gastrointestinal tract and occasionally the heart.

Juvenile Polymyositis

This is a form of inflammation of the muscles in the juvenile population.

Polymyositis

This is an entity that is similar to dermatomyositis but without the skin manifestations. It manifests itself with slow progressive muscle weakness, whereby lifting arms and even combing one's hair, as well as climbing steps and getting out of a chair, can become difficult. Muscle pains are frequent.

Inflammatory Myopathies: This is a general term used to describe the various muscle diseases associated with autoimmunity.

Vasculitis

This is an array of numerous conditions. There is a condition most commonly manifested with skin changes, typically in the legs, which show red and purple spots that can actually be felt and as such, they are called "palpable." The term vasculitis encompasses various forms of blood vessel inflammation and can affect numerous organs. It frequently manifests itself with joint pain and muscle pain, as well as numbness, weakness, and feelings of pins and needles.

The conditions can involve the kidneys, lungs, paranasal sinuses and the eyes. Surprisingly, the diagnosis is occasionally made by an ear, nose and throat specialist when there is chronic sinus change, especially manifested by ulcerations in the nasal septum. Additionally, there are numerous subjective presentations of fever, fatigue, weight loss, and generalized aches and pains. The exact organs that are involved require extensive laboratory and imaging studies, and occasional biopsies.

Psoriatic arthritis

As the name implies, this is an arthritic condition associated with psoriasis. The clinical manifestations are pain and joint swelling in the toes, wrists, ankles, and fingers. Very peculiarly, the toe inflammatory manifestations are characterized as "sausage-like," which makes the swelling characteristic of this condition. The condition can sometimes be associated with stiffness and pain in the lower back, as well as in the hips and neck. Given the systemic nature of this condition, malaise, fatigue and even low-grade fevers can occur. Unlike rheumatoid arthritis, psoriatic arthritis is frequently non-symmetrical.

Juvenile idiopathic arthritis

This is, fortunately, a rare disease. It affects young children and is manifested by swelling, warmth, pain and limitation of motion in the joints. There is generally asymmetry to the joints involved, unlike with adult rheumatoid arthritis. As a result of the condition, these children can experience growth disturbance and limb length discrepancy. The most common joints that are involved are the knees, ankles, wrists and elbows. They can also have small joint involvement, such as the hands and feet. This condition is frequently associated with a characteristic rash, which is described as salmon-colored. The care takers will frequently report fatigue, malaise and occasional fevers.

The most concerning complication is uveitis, an inflammatory eye condition, which needs to be treated aggressively. As such, all children with this condition need to be evaluated by an ophthalmologist on a regular basis to prevent severe visual loss. There are children who have inflammation of the tendons that insert into the joints, a condition called enthesitis. During the taking of the history, which is usually obtained primarily from the caretakers, it should be noted that the outlook for these children is variable. There are some in whom the condition goes into total remission spontaneously, while others have a persistent, active disease.

Ankylosing spondylitis and non-radiographic axial spondyloarthropathy

Unlike what is known as degenerative arthritis of the spine, the characteristic of this set of inflammatory spinal diseases is that it actually gets worse with inactivity, as opposed to spine disc disease, which gets worse with activity and improves with inactivity. It frequently wakes people up at night. Patients will complain of chronic low back pain and stiffness. They may also have pain in the hips. They are prone to having issues with uveitis in the eyes, which need to be addressed quickly. Since this is a systemic illness, they will frequently complain of fatigue and loss of appetite. Occasionally, psoriasis is associated with these conditions. It should be noted that the differential diagnosis of spinal arthritis is sometimes difficult to accomplish. The history may not be sufficient to differentiate this condition from the classical, so-called degenerative spinal arthritis cases. As such, laboratory testing for HLA B27, ESR, CRP and imaging studies searching for inflammatory disease needs to be accomplished as early as possible.

Inflammatory eye disease

The manifestations of inflammation of the eyes can vary from blurred vision to eye pain and redness, as well as photophobia, which means sensitivity to light. Generally, these conditions are cared for by the ophthalmologists. However, there are situations in which the ophthalmologist would prefer a rheumatologist to handle biologic agents, given the fact that rheumatologists are frequently more familiar with these agents.

Crystal synovitis

The two conditions associated with this crystal synovitis are gout and pseudogout.

They most commonly present with acute, single-joint inflammation and pain. Gout is frequently associated with severe pain in the great toe. When taking a good history, one should search for recent dietary indiscretion, whereby the individual will have recently had foods that are high in purines, which are the precursors of uric acid in the body. The most common foods are red meats, legumes, seafood, and organ meats such as liver. Another culprit in dietary intake is alcohol, which, in and of itself, does not have purines but causes the body to raise uric acid levels abruptly. The peculiar aspect of gouty attacks is that an attack of severe gout frequently occurs in the presence of a sudden change in the uric acid levels in the blood. This change in uric acid levels can be either a sudden rise or a sudden lowering of the uric acid levels. As such, in taking a history, one should look for environmental changes that might have altered the uric acid level in that person, which could include recent uric acid-lowering medications or dietary indiscretion. The fact that a sudden lowering of the uric acid can generate an attack is counterintuitive, but very important to understand in terms of understanding and treating gout.

A major challenge in gouty arthropathy is the presence of uric acid deposits, known as tophi. The presence of these deposits creates a number of issues. They act as a reservoir for uric acid and make lowering uric acid levels in the blood difficult, and prevent decreasing the number of gouty attacks given their presence. Additionally, they can present pressure points, making it difficult to wear shoes and other areas of discomfort. Finally, the tophi can actually open up and become infected, which creates a real issue given the difficulty of antibiotics to penetrate these tophi. Kidney stones are also a potential possibility and potential risk given the possibility of the uric acid causing the stones.

Arthritis caused by infection

This is an area where the rheumatologist plays a major role, not so much in terms of treatment but rather in suspicion of the diagnosis. When the history is murky, one should always consider the possibility of an infectious joint. When there is a suspicion of joint infection, it should be considered an emergency, and the appropriate diagnostic maneuvers, such as removing the synovial fluid for analysis and starting antibiotics, are imperative to prevent permanent damage. Most commonly, this needs the assistance of an infectious disease consultant.

A relatively rare but peculiar condition called reactive arthritis can occur, resulting from an infection elsewhere in the body, not in the joint. In this condition, the body responds with an arthritic manifestation. Salmonella, which is caused by contaminated food, surprisingly, can result in joint inflammation occurring a few weeks after exposure to the Salmonella. As such, the history should include a search for previous food-induced bowel changes.

Lyme disease is not truly an infectious disease but rather a response to exposure to a tick bite when the tick carries a bacterium called spirochete. In this instance, getting a good history is essential. There needs to be a search for exposure to a tick bite and frequently for a rash called bullseye rash resulting from the bite. Individuals will frequently describe fever, fatigue, headaches and musculoskeletal pains. It should be noted that neurological manifestations, especially facial paralysis and severe headaches, can occur. The joints most commonly involved are the large joints, such as the knees. In rare cases, there are cardiac issues as well. When a person comes in with Bell's palsy, a search for Lyme disease is imperative.

Chapter 6

The complex therapeutic intervention and treatment of the various arthritic/rheumatic illnesses

Since I originally started practicing rheumatology some six decades ago, there has been a dramatic change in how treatment is viewed. From my perspective, the advent of treatment guidelines is positive in terms of focusing on the appropriate therapeutic intervention. However, I believe that guidelines have the potential of being used in place of clinical judgment. Every human being is different. Every illness is different. Broad guidelines do not help the particular individual who is seeking help.

We are currently living in an age of digitalization, where everything needs to have a number. An example of this is measuring pain. The patient is confronted with a question of how painful the problem is on a scale of 1 to 10. Needless to say, we are all familiar with the variable approach and response individuals have to pain. There are those who will not tolerate any pain, while there are others for whom pain can be tolerated at great levels. As such, there will be one individual who will call a minor pain 9, while others are very stoic and report a 2 for severe pain.

The choice of therapeutic intervention must be highly individualized. It must take into account the objective and internal feelings of the patient, the potential for permanent damage, the risks involved in treatment and the overall clinical picture presented in each individual case. Guidelines should only be guidelines. They should not be the final determination of therapeutic intervention.

Treatment options in Rheumatoid Arthritis

I must preface this section by explaining that I have generally listed the medications by the brand name because they are easier to pronounce and read, and this is not to be taken as an endorsement. Numerous biosimilars are now on the market.

This section describes my feelings regarding the treatment of rheumatoid arthritis. It obviously does not make specific recommendations to any particular individual. The ultimate therapeutic recommendation needs to come from the patient and the healthcare provider.

When embarking on a therapeutic recommendation, three parameters need to be addressed.

1. The patient: Are they of childbearing age? Do they have a history of alcohol problems? Have they tested positive for hepatitis or tuberculosis? What are their personal feelings about medications? Do they have a special fear of chemotherapeutic agents? Do they have a needle phobia, whereby injections really trouble them?

2. The level of severity of the condition: Individuals with a very high CCP or rheumatoid factor have a higher risk of active disease. Are there imaging studies pointing to early erosion within the joints? How many joints are involved?? A good test is to see whether there are more than 10 joints involved, which indicates a high severity of the disease and poor prognosis.)
3. Are there other manifestations of rheumatoid arthritis besides the joints, such as lung disease, pleurisy, pericarditis or eye issues?

The decision of recommendations regarding treatment is, as such, highly individualized. Individuals in whom the condition appears to be relatively mild could be started on hydroxychloroquine (Plaquenil), which is a relatively weak therapeutic agent that carries very little in the way of risks. Periodic eye examinations are necessary to ensure that there is no deposition of the hydroxychloroquine. This is one of the few drugs that can be offered to patients who are of childbearing age, and even while pregnant. Needless to say, there are always those in whom any medication creates allergic reactions, and these potentials must be discussed prior to starting the hydroxychloroquine.

If the condition appears to have deteriorated or is viewed initially as very active, methotrexate would probably be the best option. All potential risks must be fully explained to the patient. We are particularly concerned about effects on the lungs, liver and gastrointestinal tract. Something that needs to be addressed with great concern is the potential for hair loss. Likewise, the consumption of alcohol needs to be addressed carefully.

The nice part about methotrexate in terms of its delivery system is that it can be taken orally or subcutaneously, which offers options to individuals who have trouble with the medication due to their gastrointestinal issues, or when greater efficacy is desired and the oral route may be inadequate. It also addresses individuals with needle phobia because it can be given orally. There are times when I would try leflunomide (Arava), which has many characteristics similar to methotrexate.

The next step that I would like to try is what is called triple therapy, which consists of methotrexate, sulfasalazine, and hydroxychloroquine. I am leery of trying biologics early, given the potential of a multiplicity of side effects in the long term.

When the condition warrants it, the next step is a group of medications called biologics and targeting small-molecule disease-modifying anti-rheumatic drugs. These agents are potent immunosuppressants that are generally very effective in controlling the disease, but they do carry serious potential risks, especially infections, given the fact that we are diminishing the immune system with the medication. Some agents carry a warning of possible lymphoma and cancer. The oral medications carry a warning of possible thrombosis and cardiovascular issues. All this needs to be addressed and fully evaluated before starting this group of medications. The remarkable element of these agents is the frequent, but not universal, efficacy in controlling a disease that, until their advent, was so difficult to control and could result in severe disabilities.

There are a number of biologics on the market, and there is really no objective way to choose one over another in most cases. Historically, the group of medications called tumor necrosis factor (TNF) inhibitors has been on the market for much longer than the other agents. It is of interest that certolizumab (Cimzia), which barely crosses the placenta and is hardly found in the mother's milk and, as such, is an agent that can be offered both to childbearing-age individuals and women who are pregnant or lactating.

The brand names of the tumor necrosis factor inhibitors that are commonly offered are Enbrel, Humira, Remicade, Simponi and Cimzia. Among this group, some are given subcutaneously, some intravenously, and some can be given either intravenously or subcutaneously. Numerous biosimilars of this group are available. There is no objective evidence of the superiority of one agent over another. If a particular tumor necrosis factor inhibitor does not work, it might pay to try another tumor necrosis factor inhibitor, because they all work slightly different from each other.

The next option is a group of agents called interleukin-6 inhibitors. The two agents on the market have the brand names Actemra and Kevzara. Another option is rituximab (Rituxan), which is given intravenously and addresses the B-cell lymphocytes. Rituxan is an intravenous medication that is used for both rheumatoid arthritis and certain cancers by affecting the B cells.

There is an option of a medication called Orencia, which works by blocking stimulators of T cells. A group of agents that are given orally is called J kinase inhibitors. The brand names of those are Xeljanz, Rinvoq and Olumiant. These drugs have a problem in terms of their potential risks of creating blood clots, and should be given with caution to individuals who have a propensity for cardiovascular disease. There is a black box warning for infection, cancer and blood clots.

As mentioned above, I decided to name these agents by their brand name rather than by the generic name because I found the brand name to be easier to pronounce. Numerous biosimilar agents are on the market now, and the FDA has approved those and has found them to be as effective and safe as the original branded name.

Steroids, such as prednisone, need to be given occasionally to control severe flare-ups. Similarly, non-steroidal anti-inflammatory agents can be used on a needed basis, but require close monitoring. I would not be surprised if by the time this book is published, newer agents will have been offered on the market. This field of therapy is hopping and very exciting.

How I have been treating systemic lupus erythematosus

Addressing this condition is extremely difficult, given its multiplicity of manifestations. Over the years, there were those whom I had decided to just observe with no therapeutic intervention. Then there are those whose condition is extremely active and in whom therapeutic intervention needs to be done early or even immediately.

There really are no hard and fast guidelines on how to treat this condition. Some of the medications that I would use early are **hydroxychloroquine and methotrexate.** Under certain circumstances, a course of **corticosteroids, such as prednisone,** needs to be given. This needs to be administered in the lowest possible dose and in the shortest possible time because of potential risks caused by the corticosteroids. There are other options that are available and need to be given with great care in terms of potential risks. Rituxan is one of those agents that can be considered. It addresses the B cells and tries to calm down the inflammatory or immune process.

Over the past few years, some very interesting and potent medications have come on the market. **Benlysta, Lupkynis and Saphnelo** are potent agents that are now used when necessary. When to start using those agents has to be assessed purely on the basis of individual needs and conditions. There simply cannot be hard and fast rules. Numerous new agents are being evaluated, and, personally, I believe that this condition will be ultimately treatable/curable given the multiplicity of therapeutic trials going on at this time.

What treatments are available for scleroderma/systemic sclerosis?

Unfortunately, there really are no specific therapies for this condition because scleroderma / systemic sclerosis is not one entity.

Mild morphea:

This is an area that is generally treated by dermatologists. They use topical steroids, phototherapy and, on some occasions, tacrolimus.

Deep morphea, moderate to severe:
At this stage, the dermatologist generally requests that the rheumatologist get involved, given that rheumatologists are more familiar with the medications. There really are no good solutions for this. We try methotrexate, mycophenolate and occasional short-term corticosteroids.

Systemic sclerosis:
Here again, our treatment options are very limited. We try mycophenolate, methotrexate, and Cytoxan. There are now centers that offer stem cell transplants in an attempt to halt the skin thickening.

Complications

- **Interstitial lung disease:**

This is an area that should be handled by the pulmonologist. Some very exciting new therapies have come on the market that slow down the scarring of the lung tissue.

- **Pulmonary arterial hypertension:**

This is an extremely serious complication and again needs to be treated, from my perspective, at a tertiary care center.

- **Scleroderma Renal Crisis:**

This condition needs to be treated aggressively and immediately. I do not believe that there is adequate time to send to a tertiary care center. We do have therapeutic options available at a local hospital setting. The condition generally responds very quickly to what they call ACE inhibitors, such as captopril. Close monitoring of blood pressure is absolutely imperative. This condition needs to be treated by both the rheumatologist and the nephrologist.

- **Gastrointestinal issues:**

Scleroderma can affect the gastrointestinal tract by altering the motility of the gastrointestinal tract. This results in difficulties in the absorption of food and discomfort emanating from the abnormal motility of the gastrointestinal tract. Treatment is generally effective with proton pump inhibitors such as omeprazole. If that doesn't work, evaluation by gastroenterologists should be recommended.

- **Muscle and joint pains:**

This is where the rheumatologist comes in with supportive care such as low-dose corticosteroids and, occasionally, methotrexate if there is evidence of inflammation.

- **Raynaud's phenomenon**

Treatment for this will depend on the severity of the condition. Most individuals can tolerate this vasoconstriction without necessarily asking for therapeutic intervention. In more severe cases, a group of medications for high blood pressure, called calcium channel blockers, is offered. Examples of these are nifedipine and amlodipine. We try nitroglycerin topically. In conditions that get more progressive, PDE5 inhibitors are offered. An example of those is sildenafil. In some cases of severe vasoconstriction, intravenous prostacyclin analogs are given. I believe that these kinds of cases should be taken care of in tertiary care centers because I do not feel that office-based rheumatologists are capable of handling these very complex situations. Digital ulcers and severe vasoconstriction can be very serious issues.

At the end of the day, there really isn't very much that we can offer.

Treatments of inflammatory muscle diseases of polymyositis and dermatomyositis

This is another one of those conditions that requires individualization. Generally speaking, when the condition starts, corticosteroids would be appropriate, and the decision of oral versus intravenous therapy depends upon the severity of the condition. Once the condition is stabilized, the options are methotrexate, azathioprin, mycophenolate, and, where there is severe disease, especially of severe weakness or incurable rashes, intravenous IgG is an FDA-approved therapeutic option.

If things really go out of hand, Rituxan is an option that needs to be considered. There are some very serious potential risks with this medication, and it requires a great deal of thoughtful consideration before offering this particular drug.

I have not been impressed with Cytoxan.

Newer agents are now being evaluated. J kinase inhibitors of Xeljanz and Rinvoq, as well as the T cell modulator Orencia, are being studied.

When it comes to skin manifestations, I would prefer to have the dermatologist get involved for topical medications.

When the individual manifests interstitial lung disease, I would get the pulmonologist involved very quickly because there are newer agents on the market that can hopefully stop the progression of this disease.

What is of greatest concern is the presence of a higher risk of malignancy within 3 years of the onset of this condition, especially in dermatomyositis. As such, a thorough evaluation and search for underlying cancer is imperative for these patients. Additionally, screening for the development of interstitial lung disease is vital in such cases.

Finally, physical therapy is an avenue that needs to be considered to maintain strength and range of motion. All in all, unfortunately, there are no curative options, but with appropriate treatment, the condition can hopefully be controlled and stabilized.

Vasculitis

For this group of illnesses, it is imperative to make a specific diagnosis. There are numerous conditions listed as vasculitides. We can be dealing with large vessel disease, Giant Cell Arteritis, medium vessel vasculitides such as polyarteritis nodosa, ANCA-associated small vessel vasculitis, Behcet's disease, Eosinophilic granulomatosis with polyangiitis.

This set of diseases is actually undergoing dramatic

improvements in therapeutic options. Generally, we start with corticosteroids and then move on to methotrexate. It is of great interest that Actemra has been used effectively in Giant Cell Arteritis. We should be careful to search for hepatitis, which can be one of the instigators for vasculitis. Antiviral therapy would then be indicated.

There are a number of vasculitides associated with an antibody called ANCA. These can be very serious and even life-threatening. They require high doses of corticosteroids and may frequently be placed on Rituxan.

Very exciting is the fact that we now have evidence that the Interleukin-5 inhibitor Mepolizumab is effective in eosinophilic granulomatosis. Another area where there is much excitement is the efficacy of a drug called Otezla, which is oral and has a totally different mechanism of action from all the other medications mentioned so far. It is indicated for Behcet's disease.

It is obvious that this book cannot specify treatment for the various vasculitides conditions. However, the exciting part is that there are some unexpected, effective therapies that are being evaluated at this very moment.

Psoriatic arthritis

This condition needs to be treated in conjunction with a dermatologist, given the multiplicity of manifestations in terms of both the joints and the skin. Fortunately, there are some very effective therapeutic options, and this condition can most frequently be controlled with these agents.

When it comes to joint issues, we initially try non-steroidal anti-inflammatory agents, which can be very effective in controlling the joint manifestations. The usual next agent is methotrexate, which has been used for many years and is frequently very effective. Arava and sulfasalazine are agents that are frequently used as first-line treatments.

Fortunately, there are multiple biologics that can be tried. Usually, the first line of therapy is the TNF inhibitors, which were outlined above in the rheumatoid arthritis section. There is a group of drugs called Interleukin-17 inhibitors, such as Bimzelx, Cosentyx and Taltz. Then there are Interleukin-23 inhibitors, like Skyrizi and Tremfya. Stelara blocks IL-12 and IL-23. Biosimilars are available for many of the above drugs.

Overall, there has never been hard evidence of superiority in terms of efficacy or safety when comparing the various therapeutic options. A medication called Otezla, given orally, works by a totally different mechanism of action and is technically not a biologic. Its side effects generally involve the gastrointestinal tract. However, very surprisingly, it can affect depression adversely. The dermatologist may elect to use topical agents to calm down the rash.

What is interesting but frustrating is that the choice of a particular agent is purely dependent on trial and error. What works for patient X may not work for patient Y and vice versa. Unfortunately, we do not have a tool that will predict which agent will be effective for any particular individual.

Juvenile idiopathic arthritis

This is an area that is very exciting because of the efficacy of some of the medications available for this condition. The IL-1 inhibitors Kineret and Canakinumab can, on occasion, show dramatic improvements. We generally try the more traditional agents of nonsteroidal anti-inflammatory agents: methotrexate, Arava, and sulfasalazine. Other options are TNF inhibitors and, more recently, the IL-6 inhibitor Actemra has been approved for this condition. Other biologics are in the testing stages.

The very fact that we are closing in on a more specific line of therapies is, of course, extremely interesting and exciting. It is absolutely necessary, however, to make sure that the ophthalmologist gets involved to rule out underlying eye inflammation.

Ankylosing spondylitis/ non-radiographic axial spondyloarthritis

Life has changed for individuals with this diagnosis. When I first started out in medicine and specifically rheumatology, we used to see terrible spinal deformities emanating from this condition. With the advent of the newer agents, and provided we get the diagnosis early with treatment, the outlook for this condition has improved markedly. We generally start out with nonsteroidal anti-inflammatory agents and physical therapy. If that does not work, we start with the TNF inhibitors. Another option is IL-17 inhibitors, like Bimzelx,

Cosentyx and Taltz. Recently, J kinase inhibitors have been tried with success. I generally do not prescribe methotrexate or sulfasalazine for these patients. Occasionally, local steroid injections are necessary. Physical activity, including physical therapy, is absolutely necessary to prevent permanent spinal aberration.

Inflammatory eye disease

The most important role that the rheumatologist plays in this instance is to have a high level of suspicion of the case. There are those in whom the condition is such that there are very few, if any, symptoms. However, the inflammatory component can cause damage. Ultimately, it will be the ophthalmologist who will call the recommended medications and treatment program. There may be times when the ophthalmologist would feel more comfortable having a rheumatologist administer the biologics, given the fact that the rheumatologist has, generally speaking, more experience with these treatments.

Crystal synovitis—Gout and pseudogout

Gout has afflicted mankind for thousands of years. Historians indicate that Alexander the Great and Julius Caesar suffered from gout. It is of interest that, as far back as Julius Caesar's time, people afflicted with gout would be given a plant called Autumn crocus (botanical name is *colchicum autumnale*), whose active ingredient is today's colchicine.

Treatment of gout has to be approached from two separate avenues. On the one hand, long-term control of this disease requires control of the level of uric acid in the blood. This is generally accomplished with medications that lower uric acid levels, diet and abstinence from alcohol. Additionally, when a person actually has an attack of gout, the pain is intense. As such, the issue at hand is not to control the uric acid level in the blood but rather to control the pain. When treating a gout attack, one must take into account the counterintuitive finding that lowering the uric acid level abruptly can actually exacerbate a gouty attack. As such, lowering the uric acid level with medications generally needs to be done very slowly. The classical medications for lowering uric acid level are Allopurinol, Benemid and Uloric (flebuxostat). Under certain circumstances, when the uric acid level cannot be controlled, intravenous Krystexxa can be given, which lowers the uric acid level very quickly.

Additionally, dietary recommendations are crucial. High purine diets must be curtailed in this condition. This generally consists of red meats, legumes, anchovies and sardines, or organ meats such as liver. Additionally, alcohol can raise uric acid levels and, as such, needs to be avoided.

An acute gouty attack is extremely uncomfortable and painful. What has been generally given for them is anti-inflammatory agents, especially indomethacin. Corticosteroid injections may need to be given. Occasionally, painkillers must be offered, given the severity of this condition. The classical drug for an acute case of gout is colchicine. This drug needs to be given carefully due to potential ill effects and should never be given in very high dosages per day.

Pseudogout is not dependent upon uric acid levels. The exact cause of pseudogout is not clear, but there is evidence of calcium deposition in the cartilage, which is responsible for the shedding of crystals, which in turn cause these terrible pseudogout attacks. No specific dietary intervention is necessary. Treatment is generally symptomatic. They do respond to colchicine, but it's not as effective as in true gout. Corticosteroids and painkillers are the main therapeutic options.

Sjogren's syndrome

The treatment of this condition varies depending on the individual manifestations of this condition. We generally recommend artificial tears and occasional ophthalmologic surgical intervention for occlusion of the punctal ducts. Oral medications are pilocarpine and cevimeline, which address the dryness. Medications that address the systemic nature of this condition are Plaquenil, methotrexate, Arava and Cytoxan. In severe cases, Rituxan can be considered. A number of biologics are being tested at this time for the treatment of severe cases.

Fibromyalgia/fatigue syndrome

Unfortunately, no real good therapeutic options exist for this condition. The most important thing the healthcare provider can offer is supportive care and understanding of the debilitating nature manifested by this condition. The fatigue can be, on occasion, so severe that people simply cannot get out of bed. The medications approved by the FDA for fibromyalgia, as far as I'm concerned, do not address the actual condition, and as such, I do not believe they are very effective.

FINAL CHAPTER: WHERE DO WE GO FROM HERE?

I have been a rheumatologist since 1965. I have seen tremendous forward motion in the understanding and treatment of musculoskeletal and autoimmune diseases. The real issue, however, is that all we do at this time is treat. We don't prevent or cure. We really don't understand what causes autoimmunity. How does the body misinterpret its own organs as threatening foreign agents?

Personally, I believe that there is some agent out in the environment that triggers this entire paradigm. It may well be that the agent has not even been named by scientists at this time. If we look at Louis Pasteur, he suspected an agent, which he called the filterable agent, that could not be seen under the microscope and was clearly not a bacterium. In retrospect, he was evaluating and working with viruses. Could there be agents in the year 2026 that we cannot discern, which, in a few years, may turn out to be the culprit causing autoimmunity?

Deep down in my mind, I have a suspicion of an agent called Prion, which is very difficult to characterize. It causes mad cow disease and a condition called Kuru in cannibals in Papua New Guinea. It is also the agent responsible for a condition called Creutzfeldt-Jakob disease. The prion is more primitive than a virus in that it is a protein that is misfolded. It doesn't even have DNA and RNA. Who knows? This is pure speculation on my part.

From my perspective, the most crucial element in dealing with autoimmune diseases remains maintaining an open mind. There should be no possible explanation that cannot be tested. At the beginning of this book, I wrote a chapter pointing out the numerous unexpected and surprising findings over the years, which allowed us to gain insight into autoimmune and rheumatic illnesses. You never know where the solution will come from.

Despite the multiple limitations, my experience has been an absolute delight. I've had the privilege of observing the field of rheumatology from the early days, an unknown array of conditions with no specific names or characterization, through today, when the characterization has been established, and numerous therapeutic options have changed the entire picture of these conditions. At this time, I would like to thank all my teachers and patients who, over the years, have guided me, and with whom I have hopefully worked appropriately. Finally, of course, I must thank my wife, who tolerated years and years of intense responsibilities in various difficult environments.

I am looking forward to writing another book at a time when all illnesses will have been eradicated.

Contact information

Email address: 18abecker1@gmail.com

www.ingramcontent.com/pod-product-compliance
Lightning Source LLC
LaVergne TN
LVHW022015200926
848481LV00007B/2399
* 9 7 9 8 9 0 2 2 3 4 6 9 2 *